COMPLETE GUIDE TO COLORECTAL CANCER

Comprehensive Handbook To Diagnosis, Treatment, Prevention Strategies, Survivorship Insights For Patients And Caregivers

DEHART HAIRSTON

DISCLAIMER

This book's content is only intended for general informative purposes. At the time of writing, the author has taken every precaution to guarantee that the material is correct and current. Nevertheless, the author disclaims all explicit and implicit representations and guarantees about the availability, appropriateness, correctness, completeness, and usefulness of the material on these pages.

Since the author is not a licensed medical practitioner, the material in this book shouldn't be interpreted as medical advice. Before making any modifications to their diet, exercise regimen, or medical treatment, readers are urged to speak with a licensed healthcare provider.

Moreover, the author has no connection to any of the businesses, organizations, or people that are discussed in this book. Any mentions of goods, services, businesses, or people are purely informative and do not indicate endorsement or suggestion.

This book's content is entirely dependent on the author's expertise, study, and comprehension of the topic. Despite having taken reasonable care to offer correct information, the author disclaims all liability for any mistakes or omissions in the material as well as for any losses, harm, or damages resulting from using the information.

It is recommended that readers use their own judgment and discretion when applying the knowledge in this book to their own situations. The use or implementation of any material in this book may result in unfavorable repercussions, directly or indirectly, for which the author assumes no liability.

By reading this book, you agree to release and hold the author harmless from any claims, losses, liabilities, costs, or expenditures resulting from or related to the use of the information you get from it.

Table of Contents

ABOUT THIS BOOK

"Colorectal Cancer" is more than simply a book; it is a thorough guide that can save lives while also alleviating the worries and uncertainties associated with colorectal cancer. In today's environment, when this condition is tragically common, knowing all aspects of it is critical. This book is essential for anybody, whether they are patients, caregivers, or just concerned citizens.

Chapter after chapter, this book looks into the complexities of colorectal cancer. From the very basics in Chapter 1, which explains what colorectal cancer is, to the complexities of diagnosis, staging, and prognosis in subsequent chapters, readers are equipped with essential knowledge that allows them to navigate medical jargon and better understand their condition.

The treatment options described in Chapter 4 provide vital insights into the many techniques available, including surgery, chemotherapy, radiation therapy, and new targeted medicines and immunotherapies. This information not only assists people in making educated choices but also facilitates talks with healthcare practitioners, guaranteeing a collaborative approach to treatment.

Furthermore, this book goes beyond therapy and discusses lifestyle adjustments, supportive care, and techniques for controlling recurrence and metastasis. Chapter 7 provides practical recommendations on food, exercise, and coping methods, all of which contribute to general well-being during and after treatment.

Perhaps one of the most important portions is Chapter 9, which focuses on prevention and early detection. This book inspires people to take proactive efforts to reduce their risk and identify the illness early, when it's most curable, by highlighting lifestyle changes, screening standards, and the significance of genetic counseling.

In addition, Chapter 10 of this book looks forward to the future rather than merely the present. It delves into developing medicines, breakthroughs in screening technology, and promising areas of study, providing hope and optimism for improved results in the years ahead.

In summary, "Colorectal Cancer" is more than just a book; it's a source of education, support, and empowerment for anybody impacted by this illness. It's a must-have resource that not only informs but also encourages action, resulting in better outcomes and a higher quality of life for people with colorectal cancer.

CHAPTER 1

Understanding Colorectal Cancer

What Is Colorectal Cancer?

Colorectal cancer is a form of cancer that begins in either the colon or the rectum, both of which are digestive organs. To further comprehend colorectal cancer, consider that the colon and rectum absorb nutrients from meals and eliminate waste from the body. When cancer develops in these locations, it usually starts as little growths called polyps on the inner lining of the colon or rectum. If these polyps are not found and treated promptly, they might develop into cancer.

Anatomy Of The Colon And Rectum

The colon and rectum are essential parts of the digestive system. The colon, also called the large intestine, is a long, muscular tube that makes up the bulk of the digestive system's bottom half. Its principal purpose is to absorb water and electrolytes from undigested food, resulting in solid waste, or stool. The rectum is the large intestine's last portion, linking the colon and the anus. Its primary function is to hold feces until it is evacuated by the body during a bowel movement.

Understanding the architecture of the colon and rectum is critical for understanding how colorectal cancer begins and progresses. Cancerous cells may begin in any of these organs and, if untreated, spread to surrounding lymph nodes and other organs, making treatment more difficult.

Causes And Risk Factors

While the actual cause of colorectal cancer is not always known, several variables might raise a person's chance of having it.

The risk factors include:

• Older persons are more likely to get colorectal cancer, with the risk rising dramatically after age 50.

• Those with a family history of colorectal cancer or genetic disorders like Lynch syndrome or familial adenomatous polyposis (FAP) are more likely to develop the disease.

• A personal history of colorectal cancer or polyps may enhance the risk of future cancer.

• A diet rich in red or processed meats, poor in fiber, and missing fruits and vegetables may increase the risk of colon cancer. Obesity, smoking, and excessive alcohol intake may all contribute to an increased risk.

• Crohn's disease and ulcerative colitis, which cause chronic inflammation in the colon or rectum, increase the risk of colorectal cancer over time.

Understanding these causes and risk factors may help people make educated lifestyle choices and get the right screening tests for early identification and prevention.

Signs And Symptoms

Understanding the signs and symptoms of colorectal cancer is critical for early identification and treatment. Some typical symptoms might include:

• Changes in bowel habits, including persistent diarrhea, constipation, or stool consistency changes.

• Bright red or black blood in stool may suggest bleeding in the rectum or colon.

• Chronic stomach discomfort, such as cramping, bloating, or persistent pain.

• Unexplained weight loss and exhaustion.

• Weakness and Anemia: Symptoms of anemia, including pale skin and shortness of breath, may occur owing to blood loss.

It is crucial to remember that these symptoms may be caused by illnesses other than colorectal cancer. However, if any of these symptoms continue or worsen over time, it is critical to see a doctor for a thorough assessment and testing.

Understanding the signs and symptoms of colorectal cancer allows patients to take proactive efforts to seek medical care and perform screening tests, resulting in early detection and better treatment results.

CHAPTER 2

Diagnosis

Screening Tests And Guidelines

Screening for colorectal cancer is critical for early identification and improved treatment results. Regular tests are recommended for those over a particular age or who have specific risk factors. The most popular screening methods are fecal occult blood tests (FOBT), fecal immunochemical tests (FIT), sigmoidoscopy, colonoscopy, and virtual colonoscopy (CT colonography).

FOBT and FIT examine stool samples for concealed blood, which may indicate the presence of cancer or pre-cancerous polyps. Sigmoidoscopy examines the lower section of the colon using a flexible tube and a camera, while colonoscopy checks the whole colon and rectum. Virtual colonoscopy generates detailed pictures of the colon using CT scans.

Guidelines often differ based on variables such as age, family history, and personal health history. For example, most experts suggest beginning regular screenings at age 50, but those with a family history of colorectal cancer may need to start sooner. It is important to contact a healthcare practitioner to identify the optimal screening plan for your specific circumstances.

Diagnostic Procedures (Colonoscopy, Ct Scans, Etc)

Colonoscopy

Colonoscopy is the main diagnostic method for colorectal cancers. During the process, a flexible tube carrying a camera is introduced into the rectum and directed into the colon. This lets clinicians see the whole colon and rectum, checking for polyps, cancers, and other abnormal tissue. If any questionable spots are discovered, the doctor may collect tissue samples (biopsies) for further investigation.

Colonoscopy is used for both diagnosis and therapy. Polyps may be eliminated during the treatment, perhaps averting the development of cancer. To reduce pain, the surgery is often performed under sedation.

CT scans

CT scans, also known as computed tomography scans, are imaging procedures that use X-rays to produce comprehensive cross-sectional pictures of the body. CT scans are routinely used in colorectal cancer diagnosis to assess the disease's breadth, including if it has spread to adjacent lymph nodes or other organs.

CT scans may assist detect the stage of colorectal cancer, which is necessary for designing an effective treatment strategy.

They are often used before surgery or other therapies to get a thorough grasp of the patient's condition.

Biopsy And Pathology Reports

A biopsy is the only technique to definitively diagnose colorectal cancer. A biopsy is a tiny sample of tissue obtained from a questionable location, usually during a colonoscopy or sigmoidoscopy. A pathologist then examines the tissue sample using a microscope to check for cancer cells or other abnormalities.

Pathology reports include specific information regarding the biopsy results, such as the kind of cancer, its stage, and other features. This information is critical in identifying the optimal course of therapy. In rare situations, further tests may be conducted on the biopsy sample to acquire more information about the cancer's molecular features, allowing treatment approaches to be tailored to particular patients.

CHAPTER 3

Staging And Prognosis

TNM Staging System

The TNM staging system is a vital subject to comprehend while studying colorectal cancer. This method aids in determining the degree to which cancer has progressed throughout the body. Let us break it down:

Tumor (T): This component of the TNM system represents the size and extent of the main tumor. It varies from TX (primary tumor cannot be evaluated) to T4b (tumor has infiltrated neighboring organs or tissues).

Node (N): This section describes if the malignancy has spread to neighboring lymph nodes. It is represented as NX (lymph nodes cannot be evaluated), N0 (no spread to neighboring lymph nodes), and N2 (cancer has spread to four or more nearby lymph nodes).

Metastasis (M): This component reveals if the cancer has migrated to other places of the body. It varies from MX (metastasis cannot be determined) to M1c (cancer has spread to distant organs).

Combining these three criteria allows physicians to identify the stage of colorectal cancer, which ranges from Stage 0 (very early disease that has not progressed) to Stage IV (cancer has spread to distant organs). Understanding the TNM staging system allows patients and healthcare practitioners to make more educated choices regarding treatment options and prognosis.

Understanding Prognostic Factors

Prognostic factors are traits or circumstances that may affect the course of colorectal cancer. These criteria are critical in establishing the prognosis and informing therapy recommendations. Let's look at some crucial prognostic factors:

Tumor Grade: The grade of the tumor indicates how abnormal the cancer cells appear under a microscope. Higher-grade cancers grow and spread faster, which affects the prognosis.

Tumor position: The position of the tumor in the colon or rectum might affect the prognosis. For example, malignancies closer to the anus may be more difficult to cure and have a different prognosis than those in the ascending colon.

Lymph Node Involvement: The presence of cancer cells in adjacent lymph nodes implies a greater risk of cancer spread and may affect the prognosis. Patients with lymph node involvement may need more intensive treatment options.

Metastasis: The presence of distant metastases, which occur when cancer spreads to other organs such as the liver or lungs, dramatically worsens the prognosis. Detecting metastases early is critical for designing an effective treatment approach.

Patient Factors: Age, general health, and responsiveness to therapy may all influence prognosis. Younger people and those in excellent general health may have greater results.

Predicting Survival Rates

Survival rates are estimates of the proportion of persons with a certain kind and stage of cancer who are still alive at a given period following diagnosis. While survival rates are calculated for large groups of individuals and may not predict individual outcomes, they may give useful information. Here's how survival rates are usually calculated:

The five-year survival rate is the proportion of patients who are still alive five years after being diagnosed. It is one of the most widely utilized methods for determining cancer prognosis.

Relative Survival Rate: This rate compares the survival rates of cancer patients to those in the general population of the same age, race, and gender who have not been diagnosed with cancer.

Overall Survival Rate: This is the proportion of persons who are still living at a certain period following diagnosis, regardless of the reason for death.

Survival rates might vary greatly based on cancer stage, therapy efficacy, and individual patient characteristics. It is important to discuss survival statistics with healthcare specialists in the context of your situation, as they may give useful information about what to anticipate and how to prepare for the future.

CHAPTER 4

Treatment Options

Surgery (Resection, Colectomy, Etc)

Surgery is one of the major therapies for colorectal cancer, which involves removing malignant tissue from the colon or rectum. The kind of surgery conducted is determined by a variety of criteria, including the cancer's location and stage, as well as the patient's general condition.

Resection is a surgical procedure in which the surgeon removes the malignant tumor from the colon or rectum, as well as a margin of healthy tissue around it. This margin is critical for removing all cancer cells and lowering the likelihood of recurrence. The damaged part is removed, and the healthy ends of the colon or rectum are rejoined.

A colectomy is a procedure that removes a piece of the colon. This operation may be required if the cancer is in the colon and cannot be treated with more conservative treatments. Depending on the degree of the cancer, a partial colectomy (removal of a section of the colon) or a complete colectomy (removal of the whole colon) may be done.

Ileostomy or Colostomy: In certain circumstances, especially when a large piece of the colon or rectum is removed, the surgeon may establish a stoma in the abdomen. This lets waste leave the body and gather in an external pouch. This treatment, known as an ileostomy or colostomy, may be temporary or permanent, depending on the unique circumstances.

Chemotherapy

Chemotherapy is a systemic treatment that employs medications to kill or prevent cancer cells from developing. It may be taken before surgery to decrease the tumor and make it simpler to remove, or after surgery to eliminate any leftover cancer cells and lower the chance of recurrence. Chemotherapy medications may be given orally or intravenously, and they are often provided in cycles to give the body time to recuperate between treatments.

The chemotherapy regimen given will be determined by many criteria, including the stage and kind of colorectal cancer, the patient's general health, and treatment tolerance. Common adverse effects of chemotherapy include nausea, vomiting, exhaustion, hair loss, and an increased risk of infection. However, developments in medical technology and supportive care have contributed to reducing these side effects and improving the overall experience of chemotherapy treatment.

Radiation Therapy

Radiation treatment employs high-energy rays or particles to kill cancer cells or shrink tumors. It may be used as a main treatment for colorectal cancer, especially in conjunction with surgery and/or chemotherapy, or as a palliative treatment to alleviate symptoms and enhance the quality of life in advanced instances.

Radiation treatment involves the patient lying on a table while a machine provides focused radiation to the damaged region. The radiation oncologist meticulously organizes the therapy to minimize harm to the healthy tissue around the tumor. Radiation therapy is often administered in daily sessions over many weeks, giving the body time to recuperate in between treatments.

Radiation therapy's common adverse effects include weariness, skin irritation or redness in the treatment region, diarrhea, and rectal pain. These side effects are often transitory and may be addressed with supportive care measures recommended by the healthcare team.

Targeted Therapy And Immunotherapy

Targeted therapy and immunotherapy are emerging therapeutic techniques that selectively target cancer cells while protecting healthy tissue, resulting in fewer side effects than standard chemotherapy and radiation treatments.

Targeted treatment medications function by interfering with particular chemicals that regulate cancer cell growth and survival. Some targeted medicines, for example, inhibit the signals that cancer cells use to divide and develop, while others improve the immune system's ability to detect and destroy cancer cells. Targeted therapy may be used alone or in conjunction with other therapies, depending on the individual's tumor features and treatment objectives.

Immunotherapy uses the strength of the body's immune system to combat cancer. These medications enhance the immune system's ability to detect and eliminate cancer cells. Immunotherapy has shown promise in treating certain kinds of colorectal cancer, especially those with specific genetic abnormalities. Immunotherapy, like targeted therapy, may be used alone or in conjunction with other therapies, depending on the patient's unique needs.

Targeted therapy and immunotherapy are both active research topics, and new medications and treatment techniques are constantly being developed to enhance colorectal cancer patient outcomes.

CHAPTER 5

Surgical Procedures

Preparation For Surgery

Thorough planning is required before colorectal cancer surgery to get the best potential result and minimize problems. Your healthcare team will provide you with thorough instructions in the days leading up to your operation. This may include food restrictions, bowel preparation, and instructions on which drugs you should or should not take before the treatment.

Bowel preparation is an important step before colorectal surgery. It entails thoroughly emptying the intestine to lessen the likelihood of difficulties during and after the procedure. To fully cleanse your colon, your healthcare professional may prescribe laxatives or enemas.

To ensure proper bowel preparation, please follow these recommendations.

In addition to bowel preparation, your healthcare team will do pre-operative testing to evaluate your general health and detect any possible hazards. These procedures may involve blood tests, imaging scans (such as CT scans or MRIs), and maybe a colonoscopy to determine the extent of the malignancy.

Emotional preparation is also essential before having surgery. It is natural to feel scared or apprehensive, but discussing your worries with your healthcare team may help relieve some of the tension. They can enlighten you on what to anticipate before, during, and after surgery, allowing you to feel more prepared and confident.

Types Of Surgical Approaches

There are multiple surgical ways to treat colorectal cancer, and the treatment chosen is determined by a variety of criteria, including the disease's location and stage, as well as the patient's general condition. The major surgical options are:

1. Laparoscopic surgery, often known as minimally invasive surgery, involves creating small incisions in the belly to introduce a tiny camera and surgical equipment. In comparison to conventional open surgery, this strategy provides for a faster recovery, less discomfort, and shorter hospital stays.

2. Open surgery involves making a single, wider incision in the belly to reach the afflicted region. This method may be essential for larger tumors or if laparoscopic surgery is not an option. While open surgery requires a longer hospital stay and

recuperation time, it is still a safe and effective treatment option for colorectal cancer.

3. Robotic Surgery: Robotic-assisted surgery is similar to laparoscopic surgery, except it uses robotic arms controlled by the surgeon to make precise motions. This method improves dexterity and vision, allowing for more precise tumor removal while limiting injury to adjacent tissue.

4. Transanal Endoscopic Microsurgery (TEM) is a minimally invasive procedure used to remove early-stage rectal cancers. It entails introducing a specialized endoscope into the anus to see and remove the tumor, without the need for an abdominal incision.

Your surgeon will decide the surgical technique depending on characteristics such as tumor size, location, and general health.

Recovery And Postoperative Care

Following colon cancer surgery, effective postoperative care is required to improve healing and limit the risk of problems. Your healthcare staff will provide you with thorough instructions for recuperation, including:

1. **Pain Management:** You may suffer discomfort or pain after surgery, which may be treated with pain medicines recommended by your doctor. To avoid discomfort and improve mobility, it is critical to take these drugs exactly as prescribed.

2. **Dietary Guidelines:** As tolerated, your diet may go from clear liquids to solid meals. To reduce gastrointestinal pain and enhance recovery, follow your healthcare provider's dietary guidelines.

3. **Physical Activity:** While it is crucial to relax and allow your body to recuperate, mild exercise and walking are recommended to avoid blood clots and

improve circulation. Your healthcare team will advise you on when it is safe to resume more rigorous activities.

4. Wound Care: If you have surgical wounds, adequate wound care is essential to avoid infection. Keep the incision clean and dry, and follow any particular recommendations from your healthcare practitioner.

5. Regular follow-up visits will be organized to evaluate your healing and look for symptoms of recurrence or problems. It is important to attend these sessions and discuss any concerns or symptoms with your healthcare staff.

You may encourage a smooth recovery and improve your long-term results after colorectal cancer surgery by strictly adhering to your postoperative care plan and maintaining constant contact with your healthcare team.

CHAPTER 6

Chemotherapy And Radiation

How Chemotherapy Works

Chemotherapy is a therapeutic approach that uses chemicals to eliminate cancer cells. These medications function by targeting cells that divide quickly, which is a hallmark of cancer cells. Chemotherapy may be delivered orally, intravenously, or directly to the afflicted region. Chemotherapy aims to cure cancer, halt its spread, or treat symptoms.

Chemotherapy medications are classified into many categories depending on how they function and their chemical makeup. Some medications inhibit the cell's capacity to divide, whilst others damage the DNA inside the cell, inhibiting correct replication. Each chemotherapy treatment targets a distinct element of cancer cell growth and division.

Chemotherapy treatment regimens vary based on the kind and stage of cancer, as well as individual characteristics including general health and medication tolerance. Chemotherapy is sometimes administered in cycles, with periods of treatment followed by rest to enable the body to recuperate.

While chemotherapy is successful in killing cancer cells, it may also harm normal, healthy cells in the body, resulting in adverse consequences. These side effects might differ based on the kind and dosage of chemotherapy medications used, as well as personal characteristics. Common adverse effects include nausea, vomiting, hair loss, exhaustion, and a higher risk of infection. However, innovations in supportive care and medicine have made it easier to control these side effects, thereby enhancing the overall experience of chemotherapy treatment.

Radiation Therapy Techniques

Radiation treatment, often known as radiation, is a technique that employs high-energy particles or waves to kill or damage cancer cells. It works by targeting the DNA within cancer cells, stopping them from proliferating and expanding. Radiation treatment may be administered either externally or inside, depending on the location and size of the tumor.

External beam radiation treatment is the most prevalent kind of radiation therapy, in which radiation beams are directed from outside the body toward the tumor. Advanced imaging tools, such as CT scans and MRI, are utilized to accurately target the tumor while minimizing harm to healthy tissue. This method permits greater doses of radiation to be administered directly to the tumor, enhancing its efficacy.

Internal radiation treatment, also known as brachytherapy, involves inserting radioactive material into or around the tumor. This enables a highly concentrated dosage of radiation to be administered directly to cancer cells while sparing surrounding healthy tissue. Brachytherapy is often utilized for malignancies situated deep inside the body or tumors that are resistant to external radiation therapy.

Radiation treatment is often provided in a series of sessions known as fractions. The overall radiation dosage and number of fractions are determined by the kind and stage of cancer, as well as individual characteristics. Treatment planning is critical to ensuring that radiation is properly administered to the tumor while causing little harm to adjacent tissues.

Side Effects And Management Strategies

While radiation therapy is an effective cancer treatment, it may induce adverse effects by damaging healthy cells and tissues surrounding the treatment site. Radiation treatment often causes exhaustion, skin irritation, hair loss, and changes in skin texture or color. These side effects are often transitory and may be treated with appropriate care and medicine.

To reduce the adverse effects of radiation treatment, patients are often given detailed advice on how to care for their skin and manage symptoms. This may involve using mild skincare products, avoiding direct sunlight, and maintaining excellent hygiene to prevent infection.

Radiation treatment may have an impact on both physical and mental well-being. Coping with the stress and anxiety that comes with cancer therapy is an essential part of cancer care. Support groups, counseling, and relaxation methods may help patients and their families deal with the emotional effects of radiation treatment.

Overall, chemotherapy and radiation therapy are key components of cancer treatment because they act together to kill cancer cells and decrease tumors. Patients who understand how these therapies operate and how to manage their adverse effects will feel more confident and empowered as they go through their disease.

CHAPTER 7

Lifestyle Changes And Supportive Care

Diet And Nutrition Recommendations

When fighting colorectal cancer, a well-balanced diet is essential. Nutrient-dense meals may assist your body deal with therapy and promote recovery. Eat lots of fruits, veggies, healthy grains, and lean meats. These foods include critical vitamins, minerals, and antioxidants that benefit your immune system and general health.

Staying hydrated is also crucial, so drink lots of water throughout the day. Adequate hydration may help avoid constipation, which is a frequent side effect of several cancer medications. Limit your consumption of processed foods, sugary snacks, and high-fat meals, which may all lead to inflammation and digestive troubles.

During therapy, you may encounter changes in appetite or taste preferences. Experiment with various meals and tastes to see what works best for you. Small, regular meals or snacks might be more digestible than big meals, particularly if you're feeling nauseated or vomiting.

If you're having trouble maintaining a balanced diet due to medication side effects like mouth sores or difficulty swallowing, speak with your doctor. They may provide advice and may suggest dietary supplements or nutritional drinks to ensure you obtain the nutrients your body needs.

Exercise And Physical Activity

Staying active throughout colon cancer treatment may be difficult, but it is critical for your overall health. Regular exercise may help to decrease tiredness, enhance mood, and boost strength and flexibility.

Aim for 30 minutes of moderate-intensity activity most days of the week, such as walking, swimming, or cycling.

If you are experiencing treatment-related side effects such as weakness or discomfort, change your workout program appropriately. Consider integrating gentle exercises like yoga or tai chi that promote flexibility and relaxation. Always listen to your body and avoid pushing yourself too hard, particularly during times of exhaustion or low energy.

In addition to regular exercise, seek for ways to be active throughout the day. Take brief walks during breaks, utilize stairs instead of elevators whenever practical, and do some housework or gardening. Even tiny quantities of physical exercise may have a major impact on your physical and mental well-being.

Managing Side Effects And Symptoms

Chemotherapy, radiation therapy, and surgery may all have side effects that affect your quality of life when treating colorectal cancer. Fatigue, nausea, diarrhea, and changes in bowel habits are some of the most common adverse effects. It is important to talk honestly with your healthcare team about any symptoms you are having, as they may provide useful solutions for managing side effects.

Anti-nausea medications, laxatives, and pain painkillers may be administered to treat particular symptoms. Dietary modifications, such as limiting hot meals or increasing fiber intake, may also assist with digestive disorders including diarrhea and constipation. Furthermore, using relaxation methods like deep breathing or meditation may help decrease stress and enhance general well-being.

Supportive care services, such as palliative care or integrative medicine, may help patients manage physical symptoms and improve their quality of life. Aside from medical therapy, these programs address the emotional, spiritual, and social elements of living with cancer.

Support Groups And Counseling

A colon cancer diagnosis may be emotionally difficult, and you may find it beneficial to connect with people who have gone through similar situations. Support groups provide a secure environment in which you may discuss your thoughts and emotions, ask questions, and get support from peers who understand what you are going through.

In addition to in-person support groups, several organizations provide online forums or virtual support networks that allow you to interact with others from the comfort of your own home. These platforms provide you the ability to obtain help and information at any time, regardless of your location or schedule.

Individual counseling or therapy may also help you cope with the emotional effects of cancer. A qualified therapist can help you negotiate emotions of anxiety, despair, or terror, as well as create effective stress management skills. If you're suffering emotionally, don't hesitate to contact your healthcare team; they can link you with resources and support services to help you deal.

By making lifestyle changes and receiving supportive care, you may improve your quality of life and outcomes during and after colorectal cancer treatment. Remember to prioritize self-care, listen to your body, and seek assistance when you need it.

CHAPTER 8

Managing Recurrence And Metastasis

Surveillance After Treatment

After completing colorectal cancer treatment, it is critical to continue monitoring your health to detect any symptoms of recurrence or metastasis early. Your healthcare team will normally develop a surveillance strategy that is customized to your unique needs, which may include frequent check-ups, imaging exams, and blood testing.

During surveillance, your healthcare professional will continuously watch for any indications or symptoms of cancer recurrence or spread. This may include regular physical examinations, blood tests to detect tumor markers, and imaging procedures such as CT scans, MRI scans, or PET scans.

It is important to attend all planned follow-up visits and testing as directed by your healthcare provider. While undergoing monitoring might be stressful, discovering any recurrence or metastasis early on provides the greatest chance of effective therapy.

In addition to medical monitoring, living a healthy lifestyle is essential for avoiding cancer recurrence and boosting general well-being. This involves eating a well-balanced diet, getting regular exercise, avoiding tobacco and excessive alcohol intake, and managing stress.

Remember to talk freely with your healthcare provider about any concerns or symptoms you see in between consultations. Early identification and therapy are essential for successfully treating recurring or metastatic colorectal cancer.

Treatment Options For Recurrent Disease

If colorectal cancer recurs after the first therapy, numerous therapeutic options are available, based on the location and severity of the recurrence, as well as your general health and treatment objectives.

Surgery may be an option for localized recurrences, particularly if the cancer is limited to a specific location and can be surgically removed. In certain circumstances, surgery is followed by chemotherapy or radiation treatment to eliminate any leftover cancer cells.

Systemic therapies for recurrent colorectal cancer that have spread to other organs or distant places in the body (metastatic disease) may include chemotherapy, targeted therapy, immunotherapy, or a combination of these modalities. These medicines operate by targeting cancer cells throughout the body, rather than just one tumor location.

The location and severity of the recurrence, the outcomes of any prior therapies, your general health, and your preferences will all influence the treatment decision. Your healthcare team will collaborate with you to create a tailored treatment plan that matches your specific requirements.

It is critical to assess the potential advantages and dangers of each treatment choice, including any side effects and the impact on quality of life. Open communication with your healthcare team, as well as active participation in decision-making, may help ensure that you get the best possible treatment for recurrent colorectal cancer.

Coping Strategies And Emotional Support

Receiving a diagnosis of recurrent or metastatic colorectal cancer may be emotionally stressful, and it is natural to feel a variety of feelings such as worry, anxiety, grief, and uncertainty. Coping with the emotional burden of cancer recurrence is an essential component of comprehensive cancer treatment.

Seeking emotional support from family, friends, and support groups may be quite beneficial at this time. Sharing your thoughts and experiences with others who understand what you're going through might make you feel less alone and lonely.

Many cancer clinics and organizations provide support services and resources to people experiencing cancer recurrence, such as counseling, support groups, and educational programs. These sites may provide practical knowledge, coping skills, and emotional support that is customized to the specific requirements of people with recurrent or metastatic colorectal cancer.

In addition to getting assistance from others, learning healthy coping strategies for stress and anxiety will help you feel better overall. This might be deep breathing, meditation, yoga, or participating in creative pursuits that offer you pleasure and calm.

It's also important to emphasize self-care and make efforts to preserve your physical health during cancer treatment and recovery. This includes getting adequate rest, eating a balanced meal, keeping hydrated, and doing light exercise as tolerated.

Remember that it's good to seek assistance when necessary, and to take things one day at a time. You may overcome the problems of recurring or metastatic colorectal cancer by concentrating on self-care, receiving support from others, and continuing to participate in activities that offer you pleasure and satisfaction.

CHAPTER 9

Prevention And Early Detection

Lifestyle Modifications To Lower Risk

Making lifestyle changes may greatly lower your chance of acquiring colorectal cancer. One of the most important factors is eating a nutritious diet. A diet high in fruits, vegetables, and whole grains, with less red and processed meats, may reduce the risk. Additionally, lowering alcohol use and stopping smoking might help to maintain a healthy colon.

Regular physical exercise is another important aspect of prevention. Participating in at least 30 minutes of moderate exercise most days of the week will help you maintain a healthy weight and enhance your colon health. Obesity is a recognized risk factor for colorectal cancer, thus weight management via diet and exercise is essential.

Furthermore, people should try to minimize their use of sugary beverages and processed meals, which may lead to weight gain and an increased risk of getting colorectal cancer. Drinking enough water and keeping hydrated is also beneficial to general health and digestive function.

Finally, frequent bowel movements are needed. Getting enough fiber and keeping hydrated may help regulate bowel movements and lower the risk of constipation, which has been related to an increased risk of colon cancer. Overall, living a healthy lifestyle that includes a well-balanced diet, frequent exercise, and excellent bowel habits will dramatically reduce your chance of getting colorectal cancer.

Screening Guidelines And Options

Early diagnosis via screening is critical for avoiding colorectal cancer or discovering it at an early stage when therapy is most successful. Screening recommendations indicate that average-risk persons begin regular screening at age 45, but those with a family history of colorectal cancer or other risk factors may need to begin screening sooner.

There are many screening options available, each with its own set of advantages and concerns. The gold standard for colorectal cancer screening is a colonoscopy, which detects and removes precancerous polyps during the operation. Other non-invasive techniques include fecal occult blood tests (FOBT), fecal immunochemical testing (FIT), and stool DNA assays.

FOBT and FIT are simple tests that detect blood in the stool and may reveal the existence of colorectal cancer or precancerous polyps. These tests are usually performed at home and involve the collection of stool samples for examination. In contrast, stool DNA testing examines stool samples for particular DNA markers linked with colorectal cancer.

Another screening technique is a flexible sigmoidoscopy, which looks for abnormalities in the bottom section of the colon. While not as thorough as a colonoscopy, it may identify the majority of polyps and malignancies in the lower intestine.

Virtual colonoscopy, also known as CT colonography, is a more recent screening method that employs computed tomography (CT) scans to provide detailed pictures of the colon. It is less intrusive than a regular colonoscopy and does not need anesthesia, although it does necessitate intestinal preparation comparable to a colonoscopy.

Individual preferences, risk factors, and medical history all influence which screening strategy is best for them.

To decide the best technique for early diagnosis and prevention of colorectal cancer, talk with your doctor about your screening choices.

Genetic Counseling And Testing

Individuals with a family history of colorectal cancer or specific genetic disorders may benefit from genetic counseling and testing to better understand their risk of acquiring the illness. Genetic counseling is consulting with a skilled healthcare practitioner who may review a person's family history, personal risk factors, and colorectal cancer concerns.

During genetic counseling, people may be tested to see whether they have inherited genetic mutations linked to colorectal cancer, such as those in the APC, MLH1, MSH2, MSH6, PMS2, and EPCAM genes. These genetic abnormalities may raise the risk of colorectal cancer and other malignancies, including

Lynch syndrome and familial adenomatous polyposis (FAP).

Genetic testing usually entails submitting a blood or saliva sample, which is subsequently processed to detect particular genetic alterations. Genetic testing findings may assist people and healthcare practitioners make educated screening, monitoring, and preventive choices.

Furthermore, genetic counseling may help people and families deal with the emotional and practical implications of genetic testing and cancer risk. Individuals with a family history of colorectal cancer should seek genetic counseling and testing to better understand their risk and take proactive measures to avoid the illness.

CHAPTER 10

Future Directions In Colorectal Cancer Research

Emerging Therapies And Clinical Trials

In the field of colorectal cancer (CRC) research, developing treatments and clinical trials provide a light of hope, presenting innovative therapeutic techniques and possible breakthroughs. These studies include a broad range of approaches, including standard chemotherapy, immunotherapy, and targeted therapeutics. Immunotherapy is a potential approach in which the immune system is encouraged to detect and fight cancer cells. Immunotherapeutic drugs, such as immune checkpoint inhibitors, have shown exceptional success in certain CRC patients, especially those with microsatellite instability-high (MSI-H) tumors.

Furthermore, targeted therapy has gained popularity in CRC treatment. These medicines try to interrupt particular biochemical processes that drive cancer development, providing more targeted and effective therapy choices. Drugs that target the epidermal growth factor receptor (EGFR) or vascular endothelial growth factor (VEGF) have shown benefit in subgroups of CRC patients, especially those with certain genetic alterations.

Clinical trials are the foundation of progress in CRC therapy. These trials assess the safety and effectiveness of novel pharmaceuticals or treatment regimens, and patients often get access to cutting-edge remedies. Participation in clinical trials not only provides possible advantages to patients but also adds to collective knowledge and advances in cancer therapy.

As CRC research progresses, tailored medicine techniques are gaining popularity. These techniques use genetic profiling and biomarker analysis to customize therapy programs for each patient, enhancing therapeutic effectiveness while reducing side effects. Clinicians may pick tailored medicines that will help each patient by detecting genetic mutations or other molecular abnormalities that are causing tumor development.

In conclusion, developing medicines and clinical trials are promising options in CRC research, providing fresh hope and prospects for patients. Researchers aspire to enhance results and, eventually, reshape the landscape of CRC therapy via continuous innovation and cooperation.

Advances In Screening And Early Detection

Early identification is critical in the battle against colorectal cancer (CRC) since it allows for prompt intervention and better treatment results. Recent developments in screening technology and procedures have aided attempts to discover CRC at an early stage when cancer is more treatable and perhaps curable.

Traditional screening methods, such as colonoscopy and fecal occult blood tests (FOBT), remain essential in CRC screening. Colonoscopy enables direct viewing of the colon and the removal of precancerous polyps, lowering the risk of CRC development. Meanwhile, FOBT detects blood in the stool and acts as a non-invasive screening technique for CRC.

In addition to traditional procedures, novel screening technologies are developing, which provide greater sensitivity and convenience. For example, fecal immunochemical testing (FIT) identifies blood in the stool with more sensitivity than FOBT, making it an important screening technique. Furthermore, stool DNA testing, which examines genetic material shed by cancer cells in the feces, has the potential to diagnose CRC and precancerous lesions more accurately.

Beyond stool-based diagnostics, advances in imaging technologies have improved CRC detection capabilities. Virtual colonoscopy, also known as computed tomography (CT) colonography, uses CT scans to create detailed pictures of the colon, enabling the diagnosis of polyps and early-stage malignancies. This non-invasive alternative to traditional colonoscopy is especially useful for people who are unable or unable to undertake invasive treatments.

Furthermore, research is being conducted to create new biomarkers for CRC screening, including blood-based indicators and molecular tests. These biomarkers can identify CRC in its early stages with high specificity, providing less invasive screening alternatives for those at risk.

Finally, developments in CRC screening and early detection show great potential for improving patient outcomes and lowering disease-related death rates. Healthcare professionals may improve detection efforts and save lives via early intervention by employing cutting-edge technology and procedures.

Promising Areas Of Research

Colorectal cancer (CRC) research is an ever-changing discipline that is always exploring and discovering new possibilities. Several interesting research topics have arisen, providing new insights and possible advances in the prevention, diagnosis, and treatment of CRC.

One such region is the microbiome, a varied collection of bacteria that live in the gut. New research reveals that changes in the gut microbiota may impact CRC development and progression. Research is being conducted to better understand the intricate interaction between the microbiome, inflammation, and CRC, to develop new preventative and treatment techniques.

Another intriguing area of investigation is the function of inflammation in CRC carcinogenesis. Chronic inflammation, as observed in inflammatory bowel illnesses such as ulcerative colitis and Crohn's disease, is a well-known risk factor for CRC. Understanding the molecular pathways behind inflammation-associated CRC may lead to the development of tailored medicines to reduce cancer risk in high-risk groups.

Furthermore, improvements in molecular profiling and genome sequencing have transformed our knowledge of CRC biology. Researchers can uncover possible therapeutic targets and create individualized treatment methods by analyzing the genetic changes that drive tumor development. This precision medicine approach has significant potential for improving treatment results and lowering the burden of CRC.

Furthermore, efforts are being made to untangle the complexity of tumor heterogeneity, to elucidate the many CRC subtypes and their distinct molecular profiles. By stratifying patients based on tumor genetic features, doctors may adapt treatment methods to individual patients, enhancing therapeutic effectiveness while avoiding treatment-related toxicities.

Potential areas of CRC research include microbiology, genetics, and immunology. Researchers aim to uncover the complexity of CRC by harnessing emerging technology and multidisciplinary interactions. The future offers enormous potential for expanding our knowledge of

CRC and improving patient outcomes throughout the globe with continuous investment and devotion.

CONCLUSION

Colorectal cancer, a tough opponent in the field of oncology, has been the focus of much study and medicinal advances. As we end our investigation into this illness, many major facts emerge, emphasizing both the progress gained and the problems that remain.

First and foremost, early diagnosis remains critical in the battle against colorectal cancer. Screening approaches such as colonoscopies, fecal occult blood tests, and stool DNA testing have shown useful in detecting precancerous polyps or early-stage malignancies when therapy is most successful. Encouraging broad use of these screening methods is critical for lowering disease-related death rates.

Second, treatment options for colorectal cancer have advanced dramatically, giving patients a better chance of survival and a higher quality of life. Surgical methods have improved, with less invasive treatments becoming more popular. Furthermore, targeted treatments and immunotherapies have transformed the cancer therapy landscape, offering individualized methods that target particular biochemical pathways or use the body's immune system to battle malignancies.

However, despite these advances, difficulties remain. Access to screening and treatment is unequal, especially in marginalized populations or areas with minimal healthcare infrastructure. Addressing gaps in healthcare access and raising awareness about the need for early diagnosis are crucial steps in the continuing fight against colorectal cancer.

Furthermore, ongoing study into the underlying biology of colorectal cancer is critical for generating new therapeutic techniques and improving current therapies. Collaboration among physicians, researchers, and pharmaceutical corporations is critical for accelerating innovation and converting scientific findings into clinical practice.

To summarize, although tremendous progress has been achieved in the prevention, detection, and treatment of colorectal cancer, continued vigilance, and collaborative efforts are essential to address the remaining hurdles and improve outcomes for people impacted by this illness. By taking a multidisciplinary approach and focusing on both scientific innovation and equitable healthcare access, we can work toward a future in which colorectal cancer is not only treated but also preventive.

THE END